The Ultimate KETO Savory Chaffle Cooking Guide

Delicious Savory Chaffle Recipes For Weight Loss

Lily Sherman

1

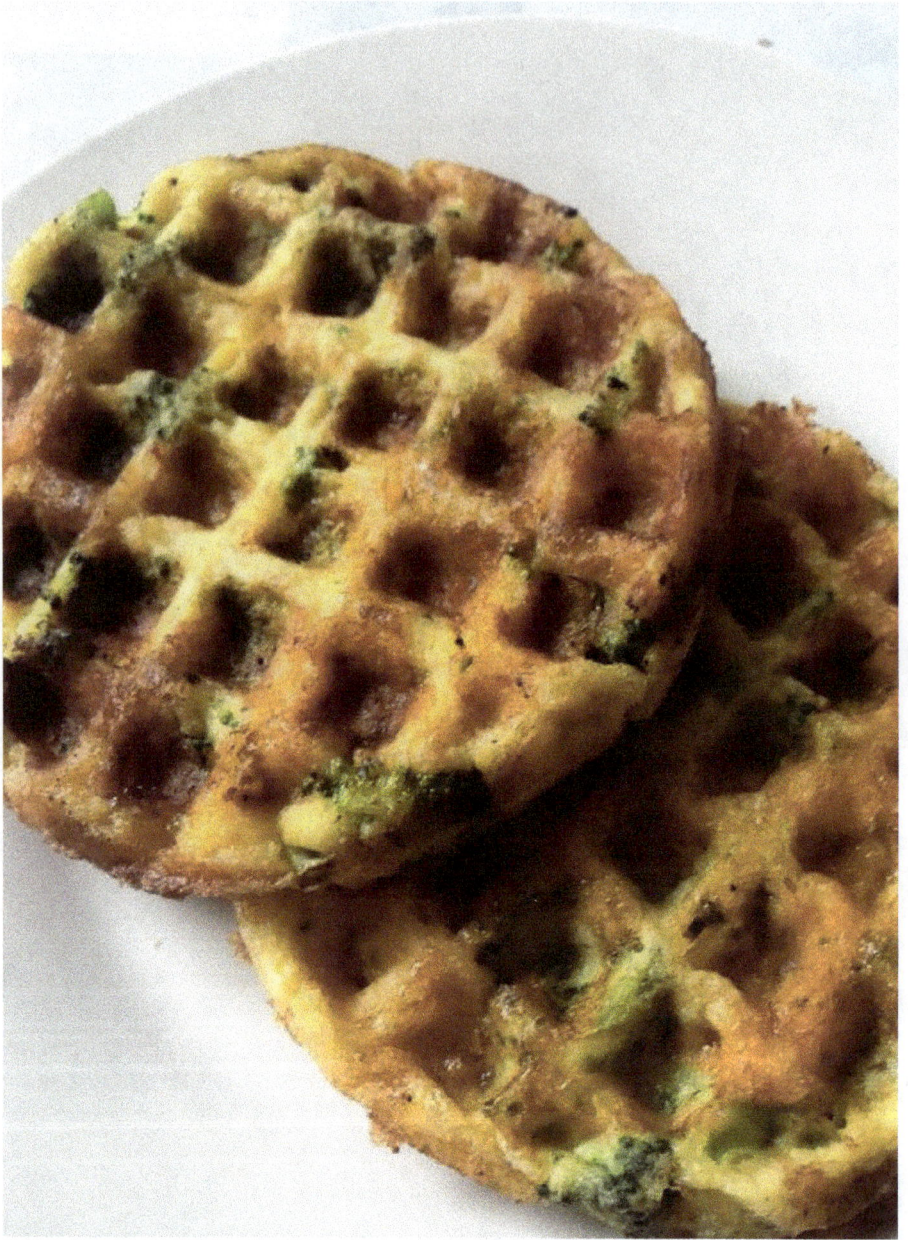

Table of contents

Chaffle Bagel

Preparation: 5 minutes

Cooking: 5 minutes

Ingredients

- 1 large egg
- 1 tsp of coconut flour
- 1 tsp of Bagel seasoning
- 1/2 cup of shredded mozzarella
- 2 tsp of cream cheese for serving.

Directions

1. First step is to pre-heat the mini waffle iron.
2. Then you whisk the egg in a bowl with the bagel seasoning, coconut flour then stir in the cheese.
3. Spread half of the egg you have mixed with the other ingredients into the waffle iron and allow it to cook for about 3 minutes.
4. Then you Remove the waffle and repeat the steps with the remaining egg mixture.
5. Next step is to spread each bagel waffle with cream cheese. You can also sprinkle additional bagel seasoning.

Bruleed French Toast Chaffle Monte Cristo

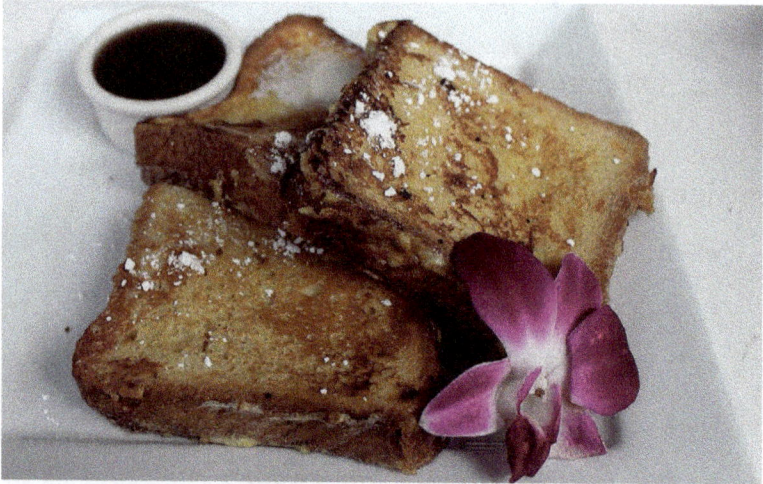

Preparation: 5 minutes

Cooking: 10 minutes

Servings: 1

Ingredients

<u>For the chaffles:</u>

- 1 egg
- 1/8 tsp baking powder
- 1/4 tsp cinnamon

- 1/2 tsp monkfruit
- 1 tbsp cream cheese
- 2 tsp brown sugar substitute

For the filling:

- 2 oz deli ham
- 2 oz deli turkey
- 1 slice provolone cheese
- 1/2 tsp sugar-free jelly

Directions

1. Preheat now your waffle maker.
2. Place all the chaffle ingredients, except the sugar substitute, inside a blender. Make sure to place the cream cheese closest to the blades. Blend the ingredients until you achieve a smooth consistency.
3. Sprinkle your waffle maker with 1/2 tsp of brown sugar substitute.
4. Onto your waffle maker, pour 1/2 of the batter. Sprinkle another 1/2 teaspn of the brown sugar substitute.
5. Close the lid and allow the batter to cook for 3-5 minutes.
6. Remove now the chaffle. Repeat the steps until you used up all the batter.

7. Prepare the chaffle by spreading jelly on one surface of the chaffle.

8. Following this order, place the ham, turkey, and cheese in a tiny, microwaveable bowl. Place inside the microwave. Heat until the cheese is melt.

9. Invert the bowl onto the chaffle so that the contents transfer onto the chaffle. The cheese should be under the ham and turkey, directly sitting on top of the chaffle.

10. Top with the other chaffle and flip it over before serving.

Ham Sandwich Chaffle

Preparation: 6 minutes

Cooking: 8 Minutes

Servings: 2

Ingredients

- 1 organic egg, beaten
- ½ cup Monterrey Jack cheese, shredded
- 1 teaspn coconut flour
- Pinch of garlic powder

Filling:

- 2 sugar-free ham slices
- 1 tiny tomato, sliced
- 2 lettuce leaves

Directions

1. Preheat now a waffle iron and then grease it.
2. For chaffles: In a bowl, put all ingredients and Mix well until well combined with a fork. Place half of the mixture into Preheat nowed waffle iron and cook for about 3–4 minutes.

3. Repeat now with the remaining mixture.

4. Serve each chaffle with filling ingredients.

Nutrition:

Calories: 175, Fat: 0.9g, Carbs: 34.9g, Protein: 6.7g, Fiber: 7.5g

Chicken Sandwich Chaffle

Preparation: 6 minutes.

Cooking: 8 Minutes

Servings: 2

Ingredients

Chaffles:

- 1 large organic egg, beaten
- ½ cup cheddar cheese, shredded
- Pinch of salt and ground black pepper

Filling:

- 1 (6-ounce of) cooked chicken breast, halved
- 2 lettuce leaves
- ¼ of tiny onion, sliced
- 1 tiny tomato, sliced

Directions

1. Preheat now a waffle iron and then grease it.
2. For chaffles: In a bowl, put all ingredients and Mix well until well combined with a fork. Place half of the

13

mixture into Preheat nowed waffle iron and cook for about 3–4 minutes.

3. Repeat now with the remaining mixture.
4. Serve each chaffle with filling ingredients.

Nutrition:

Calories: 194, Fat: 3.8g, Carbs: 29.0g, Protein: 10.9g, Fiber: 9.4g

Bacon and Cheese Chaffle Sandwich

Preparation: 30 mins

Cooking: 5 mins

Ingredients

- 1 egg
- ½ cup of shredded mozzarella cheese
- 2 Tbspn of coconut flour
- ½ tsp of baking powder
- 1 teaspn of Italian herbs
- 2 tbspn of almond oil
- 1 slice of cheddar cheese
- 2 bacon strips

Directions

1. Start with a simple chaffle base. Mix in a bowl shredded mozzarella cheese, coconut flour, baking powder, Italian herbs, and an egg.
2. Whisk this mixture well. Then take a waffle machine and Preheat now it to around medium heat.

3. Once it is Preheat, sprinkle some cheese on the waffle machine. Add the mixture on top of the cheese base and top it off with more cheese.

4. Let this cook in the machine for 4 minutes until the color changes to a golden brown.

5. Then turn the heat below a pan. Then add almond oil in the pan and cook the oil's bacon strips. Take them out once they are fried.

6. Now it is time for the assembly of the sandwich. Add your bacon and cheese to the sandwich and enjoy it.

Nutrition:

Calories 449, Fat 30g, Protein 24g, Carbohydrates 2.2g

Grilled Cheese Chaffle Sandwich

Preparation: 45 mins

Cooking: 10 mins

Ingredients

- 1 egg
- ½ cup of cheddar cheese (shredded)
- ¼ teaspn of baking powder
- ¼ tsp of garlic powder
- 2 slices of American cheese
- 1 ½ tbspn of butter

Directions

1. To make the chaffle bread. Begin your preparation by mixing in a bowl shredded cheddar cheese, baking powder, and the egg.
2. Once you have mixed them thoroughly, turn your waffle machine and Preheat now it to around medium heat. Once it is Preheated, pour the mixture on the machine and close the lid.

3. The chaffle should cook for at least 3 to 4 minutes until the color changes to a golden brown. Repeat the process to have two chaffles.
4. Then take a pan and turn heat below it to medium. Place two slices of your favorite cheese (in this case, American cheese) in between two chaffles. Put butter on the pan and allow it to Melt now.
5. Once the butter has melt, add a chaffle cheese sandwich to the pan and cook each side for at least 1 minute.
6. Remove now the sandwich from the pan and enjoy your hot and tasty keto sandwich.

Nutrition:

Calories 549, Carbohydrates 3g, Protein 27 g, Fat 48 g

Ham, Cheese & Tomato Chaffle Sandwich

Preparation: 5 minutes

Cooking: 10 minutes

Servings: 2

Ingredients

- 1 teaspn olive oil
- 2 slices ham
- 4 basic chaffles (Choose 1 recipe from Chapter 1)
- 1 tbspn mayonnaise
- 2 slices Provolone cheese
- 1 tomato, sliced

Directions

1. Add the olive oil to a pan over medium heat.
2. Cook the ham for 1 minute per side.
3. Spread the chaffles with mayonnaise.
4. Top with the ham, cheese and tomatoes.
5. Top with another chaffle to make a sandwich.

Peanut Butter Sandwich Chaffle

Preparation: 15 minutes

Servings: 1

Ingredients

For chaffle:

- 1 egg, lightly beaten
- 1/2 cup mozzarella cheese, shredded
- 1/4 tsp espresso powder
- 1 tbsp unsweetened chocolate chips
- 1 tbsp Swerve
- 2 tbsp unsweetened cocoa powder

For filling:

- 1 tbsp butter, softened
- 2 tbsp Swerve
- 3 tbsp creamy peanut butter

Directions

1. Preheat now your waffle maker.
2. In a bowl, whisk together egg, espresso powder, chocolate chips, Swerve, and cocoa powder.
3. Add mozzarella cheese and stir well.

4. Spray waffle maker with cooking spray.

5. Pour 1/2 of the batter in the hot waffle maker and cook for 3-4 minutes or until golden brown. Repeat now with the remaining batter.

6. For filling: In a tiny bowl, stir together butter, Swerve, and peanut butter until smooth.

7. Once chaffles is cool, then spread filling mixture between two chaffle and place in the fridge for 10 minutes.

8. Cut chaffle sandwich in half and serve.

Chicken Chaffle Sandwich

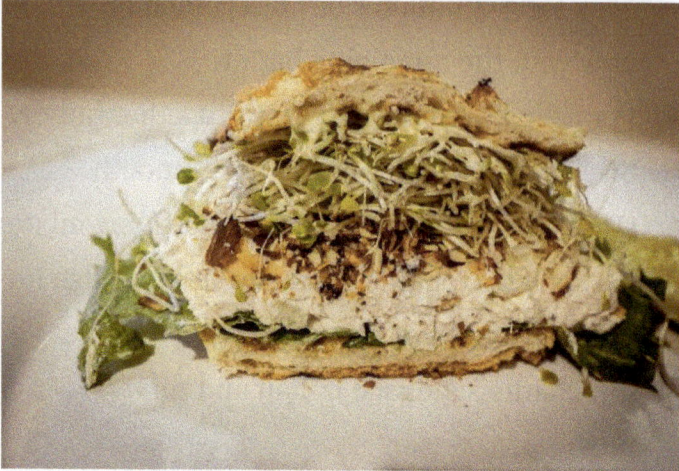

Preparation: 5 minutes

Cooking: 15 minutes

Servings: 2

Ingredients

- 1 chicken breast fillet, sliced into strips
- Salt and pepper to taste
- 1 teaspn dried rosemary
- 1 tbspn olive oil
- 4 basic chaffles (Choose 1 recipe form Chapter 1)

- 2 tbsps butter, Melt
- 2 tbsps Parmesan cheese, grated

Directions

1. Season the chicken strips with salt, pepper and rosemary.
2. Add olive oil to a pan over medium low heat.
3. Cook the chicken until brown on both sides.
4. Spread butter on top of each chaffle.
5. Sprinkle cheese on top.
6. Place the chicken on top and top with another chaffle.

Berry Sauce and Sandwich Chaffles

Preparation: 6 minutes

Cooking: 8 Minutes

Servings: 2

Ingredients

Filling:

- 3 ounce ofs frozen mixed berries, thawed with the juice
- 1 tbspn erythritol
- 1 tbspn water
- ¼ tbspn fresh lemon juice
- 2 teaspns cream

Chaffles:

- 1 large organic egg, beaten
- ½ cup cheddar cheese, shredded
- 2 tbsps almond flour

Directions

1. For berry sauce: in a pan, add the berries, erythritol, water and lemon juice over medium heat and cook for about 8– min, pressing with the spoon occasionally.
2. Remove now the pan of sauce from heat and set aside to cool before serving.
3. Preheat now a mini waffle iron and then grease it.
4. In a bowl, add the egg, cheddar cheese and almond flour and beat until well combined. Place half of the mixture into Preheat nowed waffle iron and cook for about 3–5 minutes.
5. Repeat now with the remaining mixture.
6. Serve each chaffle with cream and berry sauce.

Nutrition:

Calories: 548, Fat: 20.7g, Protein: 46g

Pork Sandwich Chaffle

Preparation: 6 minutes

Cooking: 16 Minutes

Servings: 4

Ingredients

Chaffles:

- 2 large organic eggs
- ¼ cup superfine blanched almond flour
- ¾ teaspn organic baking powder
- ½ teaspn garlic powder
- 1 cup cheddar cheese, shredded

Filling:

- 12 ounce ofs cooked pork, cut into slices
- 1 tomato, sliced
- 4 lettuce leaves

Directions

1. Preheat now a mini waffle iron and then grease it.

2. For chaffles: in a bowl, add the eggs, almond flour, baking powder, garlic powder, and beat until well combined.
3. Add the cheese and stir to combine.
4. Place ¼ of the mixture into Preheat nowed waffle iron and cook for about 3–minutes.
5. Repeat now with the remaining mixture.
6. Serve each chaffle with filling ingredients.

Nutrition:

Calories: 67, Fat: 8g, Protein: 3g, Sugar: 0g

Tomato Sandwich Chaffle

Preparation: 6 minutes

Cooking: 6 Minutes

Servings: 2

Ingredients

Chaffles:

- 1 large organic egg, beaten
- ½ cup Colby jack cheese, shredded finely
- 1/8 teaspn organic vanilla extract

Filling:

- 1 tiny tomato, sliced
- 2 teaspns fresh basil leaves

Directions

1. Preheat now a mini waffle iron and then grease it.
2. For chaffles: in a tiny bowl, place all the Ingredients and stir to combine.
3. Place half of the mixture into Preheat nowed waffle iron and cook for about minutes.

28

4. Repeat now with the remaining mixture.

5. Serve each chaffle with tomato slices and basil leaves.

Nutrition:

Calories: 285, Fat: 20.5g, Protein: 8.6g

Sloppy Joe Chaffles

Preparation: 10 minutes

Cooking: 5 minutes

Servings: 4

Ingredients

Sloppy jaw:

- 1 lb. ground beef
- 1 tsp. onion powder
- 1 teaspn of garlic
- 3 tbsp. tomato paste
- 1/2 teaspn
- 1/4 teaspn pepper
- Chili powder 1 tbs
- 1 teaspn of cocoa powder this is (optional)
- Usually, 1/2 cup bone soup beef flavor
- 1 teaspn coconut amino or soy sauce as you like
- 1 teaspn mustard powder
- 1 teaspn of brown or screen golden
- 1/2 teaspn paprika

For corn bread chaffle:

- 1 egg
- 1/2 cup cheddar cheese
- 5-slice jalapeno, very tiny diced (pickled or fresh)
- 1 tsp. frank red hot sauce
- 1/4 teaspn corn extract is optional, but tastes like real cornbread!
- Pinch salt

Directions

1. First, cooking the minced meat with salt and pepper.
2. Add all remaining ingredients.
3. Cooking the mixture while making the chaffle.
4. Preheat waffle maker.
5. Put the eggs in a tiny bowl.
6. Add the remaining ingredients.
7. Spray to your waffle maker with a non-stick cooking spray.
8. Divide the mixture in half.
9. Simmer half of the mixture for about 4 minutes or until golden.
10. For a chaffle crispy rind, add 1 teaspn cheese to your waffle maker for 30 seconds before adding the mixture.

11. Pour the warm stubby joe mix into the hot chaffle and finish!

Nutrition:

Calories: 96, Fat: 1.3g, Protein: 7g, Sugar: 4.5g

Bacon Egg & Cheese Chaffle

Preparation: 3 minutes

Cooking: 7 minutes

Servings: 2

Ingredients

- 3/4 of a chopped chess cup (I used a blend of sharp cheddar and Mozzarella cheese)
- 2 eggs (scrambled)
- 3 slices of thin bacon.
- A pinch of salt
- 1/4 teaspn pepper

Directions

1. Cut tiny pieces of bacon. Scramble the egg in a medium-sized bowl and mix salt and pepper in the cheese, then add the bacon pieces and mix now them all.
2. Preheat now your waffle iron when it is open at the proper cooking temperature and pour the mixture into the center of the iron to ensure that it is distributed evenly

3. Close your waffle iron and set the timer for 4 minutes and do not open too quickly. No matter how good it begins to smell, let it cooking. A good rule to follow is that if the waffle machine stops steaming, the chaffle will be done.

4. When the time is up, gently open the waffle iron and make sure not all of it sticks to the top. If so, use a Teflon or other non-metallic spatula to pry the chaffle softly away from the top and then gently pull the chaffle from the bottom and onto the plate after you have fully opened the unit.

Nutrition:

Calories: 154, Fat: 2.3g, Protein: 4.69g

Rosemary Pork Chops on Chaffle

Cooking: 15 Minutes

Servings: 4

Ingredients

- 4 eggs
- 2 cups grated mozzarella cheese
- Salt and pepper to taste
- Pinch of nutmeg
- 2 tbsps sour cream
- 6 tbsps almond flour
- 2 teaspns baking powder

Pork chops:

- 2 tbsps olive oil
- 1 pound pork chops
- Salt and pepper to taste
- 1 teaspn freshly chopped rosemary

Other:

- 2 tbsps cooking spray to brush your waffle maker
- 2 tbsps freshly chopped basil for decoration

Directions

1. Preheat now your waffle maker.
2. Add the eggs, mozzarella cheese, salt and pepper, nutmeg, sour cream, almond flour and baking powder to a bowl.
3. Mix well until combined.
4. Brush the heated waffle maker with cooking spray and add a few tbsps of the batter.
5. Close the lid and cook for about 7 minutes depending on your waffle maker.
6. Meanwhile, heat the butter in a nonstick grill pan and season the pork chops with salt and pepper and freshly chopped rosemary.
7. Cook the pork chops for about 4–5 minutes on each side.
8. Serve each chaffle with a pork chop and sprinkle some freshly chopped basil on top.

Nutrition:

Calories 666, Fat 55.2 g, Carbs 4.8 g, Sugar 0.4 g, Protein 37.5 g, Sodium 235 mg

Pulled Pork Chaffle Sandwiches

Cooking: 28 Minutes

Servings: 4

Ingredients

- 2 eggs, beaten
- 1 cup finely grated cheddar cheese
- ¼ tsp baking powder
- 2 cups cooked and shredded pork
- 1 tbsp sugar-free BBQ sauce
- 2 cups shredded coleslaw mix
- 2 tbsp apple cider vinegar
- ½ tsp salt
- ¼ cup ranch dressing

Directions

1. Preheat now the waffle iron.
2. In a bowl, mix now the eggs, cheddar cheese, and baking powder.
3. Open the iron and add a quarter of the mixture. Close and cook until crispy, 7 minutes.
4. Transfer the chaffle to a plate and make 3 more chaffles in the same manner.

5. Meanwhile, in another bowl, mix now the pulled pork with the BBQ sauce until well combined. Set aside.

6. Also, mix now the coleslaw mix, apple cider vinegar, salt, and ranch dressing in another bowl.

7. When the chaffles are ready, on two pieces, divide the pork and then top with the ranch coleslaw. Cover with the remaining chaffles and insert mini skewers to secure the sandwiches.

8. Enjoy afterward.

Nutrition:

Calories 374, Fats 23.61g, Carbs 8.2g, Net Carbs 8.2g, Protein 28.05g

Pork Loin Chaffle Sandwich

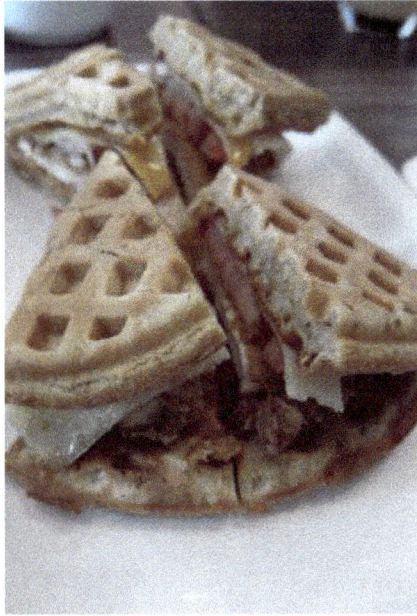

Cooking: 15 Minutes

Servings: 4

Ingredients

- 4 eggs
- 1 cup grated mozzarella cheese
- 1 cup grated parmesan cheese
- Salt and pepper to taste
- 2 tbsps cream cheese

- 6 tbsps coconut flour
- 2 teaspns baking powder

Pork loin:

- 2 tbsps olive oil
- 1 pound pork loin
- Salt and pepper to taste
- 2 cloves garlic, minced
- 1 tbspn freshly chopped thyme

Other:

- 2 tbsps cooking spray to brush your waffle maker
- 4 lettuce leaves for serving
- 4 slices of tomato for serving
- ¼ cup sugar-free mayonnaise for serving

Directions

1. Preheat now your waffle maker.
2. Add the eggs, mozzarella cheese, parmesan cheese, salt and pepper, cream cheese, coconut flour and baking powder to a bowl.
3. Mix well until combined.
4. Brush the heated waffle maker with cooking spray and add a few tbsps of the batter.

5. Close the lid and cook for about 7 minutes depending on your waffle maker.
6. Meanwhile, heat the olive oil in a nonstick frying pan and season the pork loin with salt and pepper, minced garlic and freshly chopped thyme.
7. Cook the pork loin for about 5–minutes on each side.
8. Cut each chaffle in half and add some mayonnaise, lettuce leaf, tomato slice and sliced pork loin on one half.
9. Cover the sandwich with the other chaffle half and serve.

Nutrition:

Fat 52.7 g, Carbs 11.3 g, Sugar 0.8 g, Protein 47.4 g, Sodium 513 mg

BBQ Chicken Chaffle

Preparation: 3 minutes

Cooking: 8 minutes

Servings: 2

Ingredients

- 1/3 cup of cooked chicken diced
- 1/2 cup shredded cheddar cheese
- 1 tbsp sugar-free bbq sauce
- 1 egg
- 1 tbsp almond flour

Directions

1. Heat up your waffle maker.
2. In a tiny bowl, mix now the egg, almond flour, BBQ sauce, diced chicken, and Cheddar Cheese.
3. Add 1/2 of the batter into your mini waffle maker and cook for 4 minutes. If they are still a bit uncooked, leave it cooking for another 2 minutes. Then cook the rest of the batter to make a second chaffle.

4. Do not open your waffle maker before the 4 minute mark.
5. Enjoy alone or dip in BBQ Sauce or ranch dressing!

Beef Chaffle Tower

Cooking: 15 Minutes

Servings: 4

Ingredients

Batter:

- 4 eggs
- 2 cups grated mozzarella cheese
- Salt and pepper to taste
- 2 tbsps almond flour
- 1 teaspn Italian seasoning

Beef:

- 2 tbsps butter
- 1 pound beef tenderloin
- Salt and pepper to taste
- 1 teaspn chili flakes

Other:

- 2 tbsps cooking spray to brush your waffle maker

Directions

1. Preheat now your waffle maker.
2. Add the eggs, grated mozzarella cheese, salt and pepper, almond flour and Italian seasoning to a bowl.
3. Mix well until everything is fully combined.
4. Brush the heated waffle maker with cooking spray and add a few tbsps of the batter.
5. Close the lid and cook for about 7 minutes depending on your waffle maker.
6. Meanwhile, heat the butter in a nonstick frying pan and season the beef tenderloin with salt and pepper and chili flakes.
7. Cook the beef tenderloin for about 5–minutes on each side.
8. When serving, assemble the chaffle tower by placing one chaffle on a plate, a layer of diced beef tenderloin, another chaffle, another layer of beef, and so on until you finish with the chaffles and beef.
9. Serve and enjoy.

Nutrition:

Calories 412, Fat 25 g, Carbs 1.8 g, Sugar 0.5 g, Protein 43.2 g, Sodium 256 mg

Italian Chicken and Basil Chaffles

Preparation: 10 minutes

Cooking: 7–9 Minutes

Servings: 2

Ingredients

Batter:

- ½ pound ground chicken
- 4 eggs
- 3 tbsps tomato sauce
- Salt and pepper to taste
- 1 cup grated mozzarella cheese
- 1 teaspn dried oregano
- 3 tbsps freshly chopped basil leaves
- ½ teaspn dried garlic

Other:

- 2 tbsps butter to brush your waffle maker
- ¼ cup tomato sauce for serving
- 1 tbspn freshly chopped basil for serving

Directions

1. Preheat now your waffle maker.
2. Add the ground chicken, eggs and tomato sauce to a bowl and season with salt and pepper.
3. Add the mozzarella cheese and season with dried oregano, freshly chopped basil and dried garlic.
4. Mix well until fully combined and batter forms.
5. Brush the heated waffle maker with butter and add a few tbsps of the chaffle batter.
6. Close the lid and cook for about 7–9 minutes depending on your waffle maker.
7. Repeat now with the rest of the batter.
8. Serve with tomato sauce and freshly chopped basil on top.

Nutrition:

Calories: 253, Fat: 17 g, Protein: 11 g, Carbohydrates: 21 g, Fiber: 2 g

Beef Meatballs on Chaffle

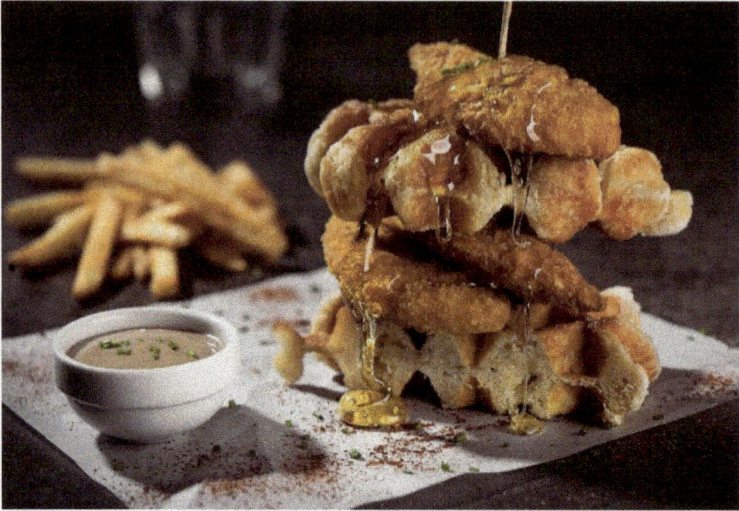

Preparation: 10 minutes

Cooking: 20 Minutes

Servings: 2

Ingredients

<u>Batter:</u>

- 4 eggs
- 2½ cups grated gouda cheese
- ¼ cup heavy cream
- Salt and pepper to taste

- 1 spring onion, finely chopped

Beef meatballs:

- 1 pound ground beef
- Salt and pepper to taste
- 2 teaspns Dijon mustard
- 1 spring onion, finely chopped
- 5 tbsps almond flour
- 2 tbsps butter

Other:

- 2 tbsps cooking spray to brush your waffle maker
- 2 tbsps freshly chopped parsley

Directions

1. Preheat now your waffle maker.
2. Add the eggs, grated gouda cheese, heavy cream, salt and pepper and finely chopped spring onion to a bowl.
3. Mix well until combined and batter forms.
4. Brush the heated waffle maker with cooking spray and add a few tbsps of the batter.
5. Close the lid and cook for about 7 minutes depending on your waffle maker.

6. Meanwhile, mix now the ground beef meat, salt and pepper, Dijon mustard, chopped spring onion and almond flour in a large bowl.
7. Form tiny meatballs with your hands.
8. Heat the butter in a nonstick frying pan and cook the beef meatballs for about 3–4 minutes on each side.
9. Serve each chaffle with a couple of meatballs and some freshly chopped parsley on top.

Nutrition:

Calories: 159, Fat: 7 g, Protein: 9 g, Carbohydrates: 15 g, Fiber: 0.8 g

Classic Beef Chaffle

Cooking: 10 Minutes

Servings: 4

Ingredients

Batter:

- ½ pound ground beef
- 4 eggs
- 4 ounce ofs cream cheese
- 1 cup grated mozzarella cheese
- Salt and pepper to taste
- 1 clove garlic, minced
- ½ teaspn freshly chopped rosemary

Other:

- 2 tbsps butter to brush your waffle maker
- ¼ cup sour cream
- 2 tbsps freshly chopped parsley for garnish

Directions

1. Preheat now your waffle maker.

2. Add the ground beef, eggs, cream cheese, grated mozzarella cheese, salt and pepper, minced garlic and freshly chopped rosemary to a bowl.
3. Brush the heated waffle maker with butter and add a few tbsps of the batter.
4. Close the lid and cook for about 8–10 minutes depending on your waffle maker.
5. Serve each chaffle with a tbspn of sour cream and freshly chopped parsley on top.
6. Serve and enjoy.

Nutrition:

Calories 368, fat 24 g, carbs 2.1 g, sugar 0.4 g, Protein 27.4 g, sodium 291 mg

Beef and Tomato Chaffle

Cooking: 15 Minutes

Servings: 4

Ingredients

Batter:

- 4 eggs
- ¼ cup cream cheese
- 1 cup grated mozzarella cheese
- Salt and pepper to taste
- ¼ cup almond flour
- 1 teaspn freshly chopped dill

Beef:

- 1 pound beef loin
- Salt and pepper to taste
- 1 tbspn balsamic vinegar
- 2 tbsps olive oil
- 1 teaspn freshly chopped rosemary

Other:

- 2 tbsps cooking spray to brush your waffle maker
- 4 tomato slices for serving

Directions

1. Preheat now your waffle maker.
2. Add the eggs, cream cheese, grated mozzarella cheese, salt and pepper, almond flour and freshly chopped dill to a bowl.
3. Mix well until combined and batter forms.
4. Brush the heated waffle maker with cooking spray and add a few tbsps of the batter.
5. Close the lid and cook for about 8–10 minutes depending on your waffle maker.
6. Meanwhile, heat the olive oil in a nonstick frying pan and season the beef loin with salt and pepper and freshly chopped rosemary.
7. Cook the beef on each side for about 5 minutes and drizzle with some balsamic vinegar.
8. Serve each chaffle with a slice of tomato and cooked beef loin slices.

Nutrition:

Calories 4, fat 35.8 g, carbs 3.3 g, sugar 0.8 g, Protein 40.3 g, sodium 200 mg

Savory Beef Chaffle

Cooking: 15 Minutes

Servings: 2

Ingredients

- 1 teaspn olive oil
- 2 cups ground beef
- Garlic salt to taste
- 1 red bell pepper, sliced into strips
- 1 green bell pepper, sliced into strips
- 1 onion, minced
- 1 bay leaf
- 2 garlic chaffles
- Butter

Directions

1. Put your pan over medium heat.
2. Add the olive oil and cook ground beef until brown.
3. Season with garlic salt and add bay leaf.
4. Drain the fat, transfer to a plate and set aside.
5. Discard the bay leaf. Cook the onion and bell peppers for 2 minutes in the same pan.

6. Put the beef back to the pan.

7. Heat for 1 minute. Spread butter on top of the chaffle.

8. Add the ground beef and veggies.

9. Roll or fold the chaffle.

Nutrition:

Calories 220, Total Fat 17.8g, Saturated Fat 8g, Cholesterol 76mg, Sodium 60mg, Total Carbohydrate 3g, Dietary Fiber 2g, Total Sugars 5.4g, Protein 27.1g, Potassium 537mg

Turkey Chaffle Sandwich

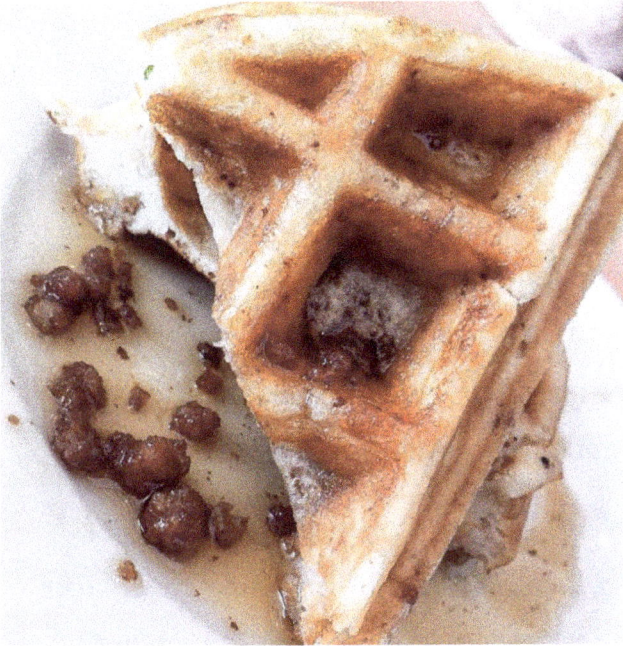

Cooking: 15 Minutes

Servings: 4

Ingredients

Batter:

- 4 eggs
- ¼ cup cream cheese
- 1 cup grated mozzarella cheese

- Salt and pepper to taste
- 1 teaspn dried dill
- ½ teaspn onion powder
- ½ teaspn garlic powder

Juicy chicken:

- 2 tbsps butter
- 1 pound chicken breast
- Salt and pepper to taste
- 1 teaspn dried dill
- 2 tbsps heavy cream

Other:

- 2 tbsps butter to brush your waffle maker
- 4 lettuce leaves to garnish the sandwich
- 4 tomato slices to garnish the sandwich

Directions

1. Preheat now your waffle maker.
2. Add the eggs, cream cheese, mozzarella cheese, salt and pepper, dried dill, onion powder and garlic powder to a bowl.
3. Mix everything with a fork just until batter forms.
4. Brush the heated waffle maker with butter and add a few tbsps of the batter.

5. Close the lid and cook for about 7 minutes depending on your waffle maker.
6. Meanwhile, heat some butter in a nonstick pan.
7. Season the chicken with salt and pepper and sprinkle with dried dill. Pour the heavy cream on top.
8. Cook the chicken slices for about 10 minutes or until golden brown.
9. Cut each chaffle in half.
10. On one half add a lettuce leaf, tomato slice, and chicken slice. Cover with the other chaffle half to make a sandwich.
11. Serve and enjoy.

Nutrition:

Calories 381, fat 26.3 g, carbs 2.5 g, sugar 1 g, Protein 32.9 g, sodium 278 mg

Bbq Sauce Pork Chaffle

Cooking: 15 Minutes

Servings: 4

Ingredients

- ½ pound ground pork
- 3 eggs
- 1 cup grated mozzarella cheese
- Salt and pepper to taste
- 1 clove garlic, minced
- 1 teaspn dried rosemary
- 3 tbsps sugar-free BBQ sauce

Other:

- 2 tbsps butter to brush your waffle maker
- ½ pound pork rinds for serving
- ¼ cup sugar-free BBQ sauce for serving

Directions

1. Preheat now your waffle maker.

2. Add the ground pork, eggs, mozzarella, salt and pepper, minced garlic, dried rosemary, and BBQ sauce to a bowl.

3. Mix well until combined.

4. Brush the heated waffle maker with butter and add a few tbsps of the batter.

5. Close the lid and cook for about 7–8 minutes depending on your waffle maker.

6. Serve each chaffle with some pork rinds and a tbspn of BBQ sauce.

Nutrition:

Calories 350, fat 21.1 g, carbs 2.g, sugar 0.3 g, Protein 36.9 g, sodium 801 mg

Pork Tzatziki Chaffle

Cooking: 25 Minutes

Servings: 4

Ingredients

- 4 eggs
- 2 cups grated provolone cheese
- Salt and pepper to taste
- 1 teaspn dried rosemary
- 1 teaspn dried oregano

Pork loin:

- 2 tbsps olive oil
- 1 pound pork tenderloin
- Salt and pepper to taste

Tzatziki sauce:

- 1 cup sour cream
- Salt and pepper to taste
- 1 cucumber, peeled and diced
- 1 teaspn garlic powder
- 1 teaspn dried dill

Other:

- 2 tbsps butter to brush your waffle maker

Directions

1. Preheat now your waffle maker.
2. Add the eggs, grated provolone cheese, dried rosemary, and dried oregano to a bowl. Season with salt and pepper to taste.
3. Mix well until combined.
4. Brush the heated waffle maker with butter and add a few tbsps of the batter.
5. Close the lid and cook for about 7 minutes depending on your waffle maker.
6. Meanwhile, heat the olive oil in a nonstick frying pan. Generously season the pork tenderloin with salt and pepper and cook it for about 7 minutes on each side.
7. Mix now the sour cream, salt and pepper, diced cucumber, garlic powder and dried dill in a bowl.
8. Serve each chaffle with a few tbsps of tzatziki sauce and slices of pork tenderloin.

Nutrition:

Calories 700, fat 50.g, carbs 6 g, sugar 1.5 g, Protein 54.4 g,
sodium 777 mg

Mediterranean Lamb Kebabs On Chaffle

Cooking: 15 Minutes

Servings: 4

Ingredients

- 4 eggs
- 2 cups grated mozzarella cheese
- Salt and pepper to taste
- 1 teaspn garlic powder
- ¼ cup Greek yogurt
- ½ cup coconut flour
- 2 teaspns baking powder

Lamb kebabs:

- 1 pound ground lamb meat
- Salt and pepper to taste
- 1 egg
- 2 tbsps almond flour
- 1 spring onion, finely chopped
- ½ teaspn dried garlic
- 2 tbsps olive oil

Other:

- 2 tbsps butter to brush your waffle maker

- ¼ cup sour cream for serving
- 4 sprigs of fresh dill for garnish

Directions

1. Preheat now your waffle maker.
2. Add the eggs, mozzarella cheese, salt and pepper, garlic powder, Greek yogurt, coconut flour and baking powder to a bowl.
3. Mix well until combined.
4. Brush the heated waffle maker with butter and add a few tbsps of the batter.
5. Close the lid and cook for about 7 minutes depending on your waffle maker.
6. Meanwhile, add the ground lamb, salt and pepper, egg, almond flour, chopped spring onion, and dried garlic to a bowl. Mix and form medium-sized kebabs.
7. Impale each kebab on a skewer. Heat the olive oil in a frying pan.
8. Cook the lamb kebabs for about 3 minutes on each side.
9. Serve each chaffle with a tbspn of sour cream and one or two lamb kebabs. Decorate with fresh dill.

Nutrition:

Calories 679, fat 49.9 g, carbs 15.8 g, sugar 0.8 g, Protein 42.6 g, sodium 302 mg

Creamy Bacon Salad On A Chaffle

Cooking: 15 Minutes

Servings: 4

Ingredients

- 4 eggs
- 1½ cups grated mozzarella cheese
- ½ cup parmesan cheese
- Salt and pepper to taste
- 1 teaspn dried oregano
- ¼ cup almond flour
- 2 teaspns baking powder

Bacon salad:

- ½ pound cooked bacon
- 1 cup cream cheese
- 1 teaspn dried oregano
- 1 teaspn dried basil
- 1 teaspn dried rosemary
- 2 tbsps lemon juice

Other:

- 2 tbsps butter to brush your waffle maker

- 2 spring onions, finely chopped, for serving

Directions

1. Preheat now your waffle maker.
2. Add the eggs, mozzarella cheese, parmesan cheese, salt and pepper, dried oregano, almond flour and baking powder to a bowl.
3. Mix well until combined.
4. Brush the heated waffle maker with butter and add a few tbsps of the batter.
5. Close the lid and cook for about 7 minutes depending on your waffle maker.
6. Meanwhile, chop the cooked bacon into tinyer pieces and place them in a bowl with the cream cheese. Season with dried oregano, dried basil, dried rosemary and lemon juice.
7. Mix well until combined and spread each chaffle with the creamy bacon salad.
8. To serve, sprinkle some freshly chopped spring onion on top.

Nutrition:

Calories 750, fat 62.5 g, carbs 7.7 g, sugar 0.8 g, Protein 40.3 g, sodium 1785 mg

Beef And Sour Cream Chaffle

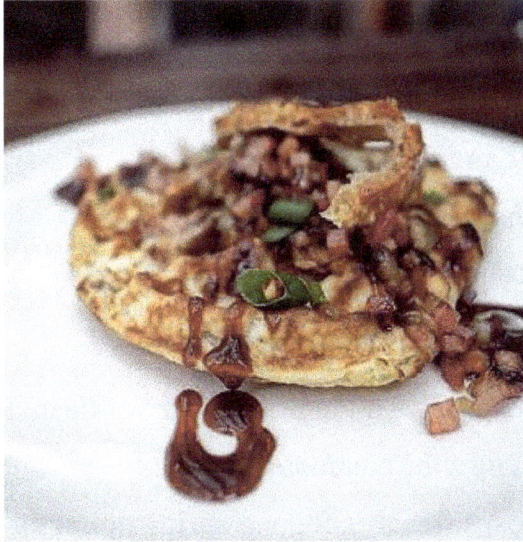

Cooking: 15 Minutes

Servings: 4

Ingredients

Batter:

- 4 eggs
- 2 cups grated mozzarella cheese
- 3 tbsps coconut flour
- 3 tbsps almond flour
- 2 teaspns baking powder

- Salt and pepper to taste
- 1 tbspn freshly chopped parsley

Seasoned beef:

- 1 pound beef tenderloin
- Salt and pepper to taste
- 2 tbsps olive oil
- 1 tbspn Dijon mustard

Other:

- 2 tbsps olive oil to brush your waffle maker
- ¼ cup sour cream for garnish
- 2 tbsps freshly chopped spring onion for garnish

Directions

1. Preheat now your waffle maker.
2. Add the eggs, grated mozzarella cheese, coconut flour, almond flour, baking powder, salt and pepper and freshly chopped parsley to a bowl.
3. Mix well until just combined and batter forms.
4. Brush the heated waffle maker with olive oil and add a few tbsps of the batter.
5. Close the lid and cook for about 7 minutes depending on your waffle maker.

6. Meanwhile, heat the olive oil in a nonstick pan over medium heat.

7. Season the beef tenderloin with salt and pepper and spread the whole piece of beef tenderloin with Dijon mustard.

8. Cook on each side for about 4–5 minutes.

9. Serve each chaffle with sour cream and slices of the cooked beef tenderloin.

10. Garnish with freshly chopped spring onion.

11. Serve and enjoy.

Nutrition:

Calories 543, fat 37 g, carbs 7.9 g, sugar 0.5 g, Protein 44.9 g, sodium 269 mg

Garlic Chicken Chaffle

Cooking: 15 Minutes

Servings: 4

Ingredients

Batter:

- 4 eggs
- 2 cups grated mozzarella cheese
- ¼ cup almond flour
- 2 tbsps coconut flour
- 2½ teaspns baking powder
- Salt and pepper to taste

Garlic Chicken Topping:

- 1 pound diced chicken
- Salt and pepper to taste
- 1 teaspn dried oregano
- 2 garlic cloves, minced
- 3 tbsps butter

Other:

- 2 tbsps cooking spray for greasing your waffle maker
- 2 tbsps freshly chopped parsley

74

Directions

1. Preheat now your waffle maker.
2. Add the eggs, grated mozzarella cheese, almond flour, coconut flour and baking powder to a bowl and season with salt and pepper.
3. Mix well until just combined.
4. Spray your waffle maker with cooking spray to prevent the chaffles from sticking. Add a few tbsps of the batter to the heated and greased waffle maker.
5. Close the lid and cook for about 7 minutes depending on your waffle maker.
6. Repeat now with the rest of the batter.
7. Meanwhile, Melt now the butter in a nonstick pan over medium heat.
8. Season the chicken with salt and pepper and dried oregano and mix in the minced garlic.
9. Cook the chicken for about 10 min, stirring constantly.
10. Serve each chaffle with a topping of the garlic chicken mixture and sprinkle some freshly chopped parsley on top.

Nutrition:

Calories 475, fat 29.5 g, carbs 7.2 g, sugar 0.4 g, Protein 44.7 g, sodium 286 mg

Beef Meatza Chaffle

Cooking: 15 Minutes

Servings: 4

Ingredients

Meatza chaffle batter:

- ½ pound ground beef
- 4 eggs
- 2 cups grated cheddar cheese
- Salt and pepper to taste
- 1 teaspn Italian seasoning
- 2 tbsps tomato sauce

Other:

- 2 tbsps cooking spray to brush your waffle maker
- ¼ cup tomato sauce for serving
- 2 tbsps freshly chopped basil for serving

Directions

1. Preheat now your waffle maker.
2. Add the ground beef, eggs, grated cheddar cheese, salt and pepper, Italian seasoning and tomato sauce to a bowl.

3. Mix well until everything is fully combined.
4. Brush the heated waffle maker with cooking spray and add a few tbsps of the batter.
5. Close the lid and cook for about 7–10 minutes depending on your waffle maker.
6. Serve with tomato sauce and freshly chopped basil on top.

Nutrition:

Fat 34.6 g, Carbs 2.5 g, Sugar 1.7 g, Protein 36.5 g, Sodium 581 mg

Chicken Jalapeno Chaffle

Cooking: 8–10 Minutes

Servings: 4

Ingredients

<u>Batter:</u>

- ½ pound ground chicken
- 4 eggs
- 1 cup grated mozzarella cheese
- 2 tbsps sour cream
- 1 green jalapeno, chopped
- Salt and pepper to taste
- 1 teaspn dried oregano
- ½ teaspn dried garlic

<u>Other:</u>

- 2 tbsps butter to brush your waffle maker
- ¼ cup sour cream to garnish
- 1 green jalapeno, diced, to garnish

Directions

1. Preheat now your waffle maker.

2. Add the ground chicken, eggs, mozzarella cheese, sour cream, chopped jalapeno, salt and pepper, dried oregano and dried garlic to a bowl.
3. Mix everything until batter forms.
4. Brush the heated waffle maker with butter and add a few tbsps of the batter.
5. Close the lid and cook for about 8–10 minutes depending on your waffle maker.
6. Serve with a tbspn of sour cream and sliced jalapeno on top.

Nutrition:

Calories 284, Fat 19.4 g, Carbs 2.2 g, Sugar 0.6 g, Protein 24.g, Sodium 204 mg

Lamb Chops On Chaffle

Cooking: 15 Minutes

Servings: 4

Ingredients

- 4 eggs
- 2 cups grated mozzarella cheese
- Salt and pepper to taste
- 1 teaspn garlic powder
- ¼ cup heavy cream
- 6 tbsps almond flour
- 2 teaspns baking powder

Lamb chops:

- 2 tbsps herbed butter
- 1 pound lamb chops
- Salt and pepper to taste
- 1 teaspn freshly chopped rosemary

Other:

- 2 tbsps butter to brush your waffle maker
- 2 tbsps freshly chopped parsley for garnish

Directions

1. Preheat now your waffle maker.
2. Add the eggs, mozzarella cheese, salt and pepper, garlic powder, heavy cream, almond flour and baking powder to a bowl.
3. Mix well until combined.
4. Brush the heated waffle maker with butter and add a few tbsps of the batter.
5. Close the lid and cook for about 7 minutes depending on your waffle maker.
6. Meanwhile, heat a nonstick frying pan and rub the lamb chops with herbed butter, salt and pepper, and freshly chopped rosemary.
7. Cook the lamb chops for about 3–4 minutes on each side.
8. Serve each chaffle with a few lamb chops and sprinkle on some freshly chopped parsley for a nice presentation.

Nutrition:

Calories 537, fat 37.3 g, carbs 5.5 g, sugar 0.6 g, Protein 44.3 g, sodium 328 mg

Chicken Parmesan Chaffles

Cooking: 8 Minutes

Servings: 2

Ingredients

- 1/3 cup of chicken
- 1 egg
- 1/3 cup of mozzarella cheese
- 1/4 tsp basil
- 1/4 garlic
- 2 tbsp tomato sauce
- 2 tbsp Mozarella cheese

Directions

1. Heat up your waffle maker.
2. In a tiny bowl, mix now the egg, cooked chicken, basil, garlic, and Mozzarella Cheese.
3. Add 1/2 of the batter into your mini waffle maker and cook for 4 minutes. If they are still a bit uncooked, leave it cooking for another 2 minutes. Then cook the

rest of the batter to make a second chaffle and then cook the third chaffle.

4. After cooking, remove now from the pan and let sit for 2 minutes.

5. Top with 1-2 tbsps sauce on each chicken parmesan chaffle. Then sprinkle 1-2 tbspn mozzarella cheese.

6. Put chaffles in the oven or a toaster oven at 400 degrees and cook until the cheese is melted.

Nutrition:

Calories: 185kcal, Carbohydrates:2g, Protein: 14g, Fat: 13g, Saturated Fat:6g, Cholesterol:122mg, Sodium:254mg, Potassium: 66mg, Sugar: 1g, Vitamin A: 3IU, Calcium: 181mg, Iron: 1mg

Turkey Bbq Sauce Chaffle

Cooking: 8–10 Minutes

Servings: 4

Ingredients

Batter:

- ½ pound ground turkey meat
- 3 eggs
- 1 cup grated Swiss cheese
- ¼ cup cream cheese
- ¼ cup BBQ sauce
- 1 teaspn dried oregano
- Salt and pepper to taste
- 2 cloves garlic, minced

Other:

- 2 tbsps butter to brush your waffle maker
- ¼ cup BBQ sauce for serving
- 2 tbsps freshly chopped parsley for garnish

Directions

1. Preheat now your waffle maker.

85

2. Add the ground turkey, eggs, grated Swiss cheese, cream cheese, BBQ sauce, dried oregano, salt and pepper, and minced garlic to a bowl.

3. Mix everything until combined and batter forms.

4. Brush the heated waffle maker with butter and add a few tbsps of the batter.

5. Close the lid and cook for about 8–10 minutes depending on your waffle maker.

6. Serve each chaffle with a tbspn of BBQ sauce and a sprinkle of freshly chopped parsley.

Nutrition:

Calories 365, fat 23.g, carbs 13.7 g, sugar 8.8 g, Protein 23.5 g, sodium 595 mg

Beef Chaffle Sandwich Recipe

Cooking: 15 Minutes

Servings: 4

Ingredients

Batter:

- 3 eggs
- 2 cups grated mozzarella cheese
- ¼ cup cream cheese
- Salt and pepper to taste
- 1 teaspn Italian seasoning

Beef:

- 2 tbsps butter
- 1 pound beef tenderloin
- Salt and pepper to taste
- 2 teaspns Dijon mustard
- 1 teaspn dried paprika

Other:

- 2 tbsps cooking spray to brush your waffle maker
- 4 lettuce leaves for serving
- 4 tomato slices for serving

- 4 leaves fresh basil

Directions

1. Preheat now your waffle maker.
2. Add the eggs, grated mozzarella cheese, salt and pepper and Italian seasoning to a bowl.
3. Mix well until combined and batter forms.
4. Brush the heated waffle maker with cooking spray and add a few tbsps of the batter.
5. Close the lid and cook for about 7 minutes depending on your waffle maker.
6. Meanwhile, melt the butter in a nonstick frying pan.
7. Season the beef loin with salt and pepper, brush it with Dijon mustard, and sprinkle some dried paprika on top.
8. Cook the beef on each side for about 5 minutes.
9. Thinly slice the beef and assemble the chaffle sandwiches.
10. Cut each chaffle in half and on one half place a lettuce leaf, tomato slice, basil leaf, and some sliced beef.
11. Cover with the other chaffle half and serve.

Nutrition:

Calories 477, fat 32.8g, carbs 2.3 g, sugar 0.9 g, Protein 42.2 g, sodium 299 mg

Classic Ground Pork Chaffle

Cooking: 15 Minutes

Servings: 4

Ingredients

- ½ pound ground pork
- 3 eggs
- ½ cup grated mozzarella cheese
- Salt and pepper to taste
- 1 clove garlic, minced
- 1 teaspn dried oregano

Other:

- 2 tbsps butter to brush your waffle maker
- 2 tbsps freshly chopped parsley for garnish

Directions

1. Preheat now your waffle maker.
2. Add the ground pork, eggs, mozzarella cheese, salt and pepper, minced garlic and dried oregano to a bowl.
3. Mix well until combined.

4. Brush the heated waffle maker with butter and add a few tbsps of the batter.
5. Close the lid and cook for about 7–8 minutes depending on your waffle maker.
6. Serve with freshly chopped parsley.

Nutrition:

Calories 192, Fat 11.g, Carbs 1 g, Sugar 0.3 g, Protein 20.2 g, Sodium 142 mg

Ground Chicken Chaffle

Cooking: 8–10 Minutes

Servings: 4

Ingredients

Batter:

- ½ pound ground chicken
- 4 eggs
- 3 tbsps tomato sauce
- Salt and pepper to taste
- 1 cup grated mozzarella cheese
- 1 teaspn dried oregano

Other:

- 2 tbsps butter to brush your waffle maker

Directions

1. Preheat now your waffle maker.
2. Add the ground chicken, eggs and tomato sauce to a bowl and season with salt and pepper.
3. Mix everything with a fork and stir in the mozzarella cheese and dried oregano.

4. Mix again until fully combined.
5. Brush the heated waffle maker with butter and add a few tbsps of the batter.
6. Close the lid and cook for about 8–10 minutes depending on your waffle maker.
7. Serve and enjoy.

Nutrition:

Calories 246, fat 15.6 g, carbs 1.5 g, sugar 0.9 g, Protein 24.2 g, sodium 254 mg

Beef Chaffle Taco

Cooking: 15 Minutes

Servings: 4

Ingredients

Batter:

- 4 eggs
- 2 cups grated cheddar cheese
- ¼ cup heavy cream
- Salt and pepper to taste
- ¼ cup almond flour
- 2 teaspns baking powder

Beef:

- 2 tbsps butter
- ½ onion, diced
- 1 pound ground beef
- Salt and pepper to taste
- 1 teaspn dried oregano
- 1 tbspn sugar-free ketchup

Other:

- 2 tbsps cooking spray to brush your waffle maker
- 2 tbsps freshly chopped parsley

Directions

1. Preheat now your waffle maker.
2. Add the eggs, grated cheddar cheese, heavy cream, salt and pepper, almond flour and baking powder to a bowl.
3. Brush the heated waffle maker with cooking spray and add a few tbsps of the batter.
4. Close the lid and cook for about 5–7 minutes depending on your waffle maker.
5. Once the chaffle is ready, place it in a napkin holder to harden into the shape of a taco as it cools.
6. Meanwhile, melt the butter in a nonstick frying pan and start cooking the diced onion.
7. Once the onion is tender, add the ground beef. Season with salt and pepper and dried oregano and stir in the sugar-free ketchup.
8. Cook for about 7 minutes.
9. Serve the cooked ground meat in each taco chaffle sprinkled with some freshly chopped parsley.

Nutrition:

Calories 719, fat 51.7 g, carbs 7.3 g, sugar 1.3 g, Protein 56.1 g, sodium 573 mg

Beef & Sour Cream Chaffle

Preparation: 10 minutes

Cooking: 15 Minutes

Servings: 2

Ingredients

Batter:

- 4 eggs
- 2 cups grated mozzarella cheese
- 3 tbsps coconut flour
- 3 tbsps almond flour
- 2 teaspns baking powder
- Salt and pepper to taste
- 1 tbspn freshly chopped parsley

Seasoned beef:

- 1 pound beef tenderloin
- Salt and pepper to taste
- 2 tbsps olive oil
- 1 tbspn Dijon mustard

Other:

- 2 tbsps olive oil to brush your waffle maker
- ¼ cup sour cream for garnish
- 2 tbsps freshly chopped spring onion for garnish

Directions

1. Preheat now your waffle maker.
2. Add the eggs, grated mozzarella cheese, coconut flour, almond flour, baking powder, salt and pepper and freshly chopped parsley to a bowl.
3. Mix well until just combined and batter forms.
4. Brush the heated waffle maker with olive oil and add a few tbsps of the batter.
5. Close the lid and cook for about 7 minutes depending on your waffle maker.
6. Meanwhile, heat the olive oil in a nonstick pan over medium heat.
7. Season the beef tenderloin with salt and pepper and spread the whole piece of beef tenderloin with Dijon mustard.
8. Cook on each side for about 4–5 minutes.
9. Serve each chaffle with sour cream and slices of the cooked beef tenderloin.
10. Garnish with freshly chopped spring onion.
11. Serve and enjoy.

Nutrition:

Calories 126, Protein 12 g, Fat 0.03 g, Cholesterol 0 mg,
Potassium 220 mg, Calcium 19 mg, Fiber 1.4g

Chicken Taco Chaffle

Cooking: 15 Minutes

Servings: 4

Ingredients

Batter:

- 4 eggs
- 2 cups grated provolone cheese
- 6 tbsps almond flour
- 2½ teaspns baking powder
- Salt and pepper to taste

Chicken topping:

- 2 tbsps olive oil
- ½ pound ground chicken
- Salt and pepper to taste
- 1 garlic clove, minced
- 2 teaspns dried oregano

Other:

- 2 tbsps butter to brush your waffle maker
- 2 tbsps freshly chopped spring onion for garnishing

Directions

1. Preheat now your waffle maker.
2. Add the eggs, grated provolone cheese, almond flour, baking powder, salt, and pepper to a bowl.
3. Mix well until just combined.
4. Brush the heated waffle maker with cooking spray and add a few tbsps of the batter.
5. Close the lid and cook for about 7–9 minutes depending on your waffle maker.
6. Meanwhile, heat the olive oil in a nonstick pan over medium heat and start cooking the ground chicken.
7. Season with salt and pepper and stir in the minced garlic and dried oregano. Cook for 10 minutes.
8. Add some of the cooked ground chicken to each chaffle and serve with freshly chopped spring onion.

Nutrition:

Calories 584, fat 44 g, carbs 6.4 g, sugar 0.8 g, Protein 41.3g, sodium 737 mg

Italian Chicken And Basil Chaffle

Cooking: 7–9 Minutes

Servings: 4

Ingredients

Batter:

- ½ pound ground chicken
- 4 eggs
- 3 tbsps tomato sauce
- Salt and pepper to taste
- 1 cup grated mozzarella cheese
- 1 teaspn dried oregano
- 3 tbsps freshly chopped basil leaves
- ½ teaspn dried garlic

Other:

- 2 tbsps butter to brush your waffle maker
- ¼ cup tomato sauce for serving
- 1 tbspn freshly chopped basil for serving

Directions

1. Preheat now your waffle maker.
2. Add the ground chicken, eggs and tomato sauce to a bowl and season with salt and pepper.
3. Add the mozzarella cheese and season with dried oregano, freshly chopped basil and dried garlic.
4. Mix well until fully combined and batter forms.
5. Brush the heated waffle maker with butter and add a few tbsps of the chaffle batter.
6. Close the lid and cook for about 7–9 minutes depending on your waffle maker.
7. Repeat now with the rest of the batter.
8. Serve with tomato sauce and freshly chopped basil on top.

Nutrition:

Calories 250, fat 15.7 g, carbs 2.5 g, sugar 1.5 g, Protein 24.5 g, sodium 334 mg

Beef Meatballs On A Chaffle

Cooking: 20 Minutes

Servings: 4

Ingredients

Batter:

- 4 eggs
- 2½ cups grated gouda cheese
- ¼ cup heavy cream
- Salt and pepper to taste
- 1 spring onion, finely chopped

Beef meatballs:

- 1 pound ground beef
- Salt and pepper to taste
- 2 teaspns Dijon mustard
- 1 spring onion, finely chopped
- 5 tbsps almond flour
- 2 tbsps butter

Other:

- 2 tbsps cooking spray to brush your waffle maker
- 2 tbsps freshly chopped parsley

Directions

1. Preheat now your waffle maker.
2. Add the eggs, grated gouda cheese, heavy cream, salt and pepper and finely chopped spring onion to a bowl.
3. Mix well until combined and batter forms.
4. Brush the heated waffle maker with cooking spray and add a few tbsps of the batter.
5. Close the lid and cook for about 7 minutes depending on your waffle maker.
6. Meanwhile, mix now the ground beef meat, salt and pepper, Dijon mustard, chopped spring onion and almond flour in a large bowl.
7. Form tiny meatballs with your hands.
8. Heat the butter in a nonstick frying pan and cook the beef meatballs for about 3–4 minutes on each side.
9. Serve each chaffle with a couple of meatballs and some freshly chopped parsley on top.

Nutrition:

Calories 670, Fat 47.4g, Carbs 4.6 g, Sugar 1.7 g, Protein 54.9 g, Sodium 622 mg

Leftover Turkey Chaffle

Cooking: 7–9 Minutes

Servings: 4

Ingredients

Batter:

- ½ pound shredded leftover turkey meat
- 4 eggs
- 1 cup grated provolone cheese
- Salt and pepper to taste
- 1 teaspn dried basil
- ½ teaspn dried garlic
- 3 tbsps sour cream
- 2 tbsps coconut flour

Other:

- 2 tbsps cooking spray for greasing the chaffle maker
- ¼ cup cream cheese for serving the chaffles

Directions

1. Preheat now your waffle maker.

2. Add the leftover turkey, eggs and provolone cheese to a bowl and season with salt and pepper, dried basil and dried garlic.
3. Add the sour cream and coconut flour and Mix well until batter forms.
4. Brush the heated waffle maker with cooking spray and add a few tbsps of the chaffle batter.
5. Close the lid and cook for about 7–9 minutes depending on your waffle maker.
6. Repeat now with the rest of the batter.
7. Serve with cream cheese on top of each chaffle.

Nutrition:

Calories 372, Fat 27.g, Carbs 5.4 g, Sugar 0.6 g, Protein 25 g, Sodium 795 mg

Beef Chaffles Tower

Preparation: 10 minutes

Cooking: 15 Minutes

Servings: 2

Ingredients

Batter:

- 4 eggs
- 2 cups grated mozzarella cheese
- Salt and pepper to taste
- 2 tbsps almond flour
- 1 teaspn Italian seasoning

Beef:

- 2 tbsps butter
- 1 pound beef tenderloin
- Salt and pepper to taste
- 1 teaspn chili flakes

Other:

- 2 tbsps cooking spray to brush your waffle maker

Directions

1. Preheat now your waffle maker.
2. Add the eggs, grated mozzarella cheese, salt and pepper, almond flour and Italian seasoning to a bowl.
3. Mix well until everything is fully combined.
4. Brush the heated waffle maker with cooking spray and add a few tbsps of the batter.
5. Close the lid and cook for about 7 minutes depending on your waffle maker.
6. Meanwhile, heat the butter in a nonstick frying pan and season the beef tenderloin with salt and pepper and chili flakes.
7. Cook the beef tenderloin for about 5–minutes on each side.
8. When serving, assemble the chaffle tower by placing one chaffle on a plate, a layer of diced beef tenderloin, another chaffle, another layer of beef, and so on until you finish with the chaffles and beef.
9. Serve and enjoy.

Nutrition:

Calories 132, Protein 9g, Carbohydrates 14 g, Sodium 112 mg, Potassium 310 mg, Phosphorus 39 mg, Calcium 32 mg